To:

From:

D1682715

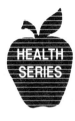

Fabulous Fiber Favorites
High Fiber Naturally

by Sue E. Willett, Home Economist

Printed in the United States of America
ISBN   1-56383-000-0

Published by G & R Publishing Co.
507 Industrial Street
Waverly, IA 50677

About the Author

Sue Willett graduated with honors from Central State University, Edmond Oklahoma, with a B.S. in Home Economics and a concentration in Business. Since 1985 she has proven her business talents as President of the M.S. Willett Co., Inc.; a leading edge company in product research, design, development and marketing.

In addition to the Health Series, Sue is author or co-author of four books and guides to healthy cooking and eating. After experiencing heart disease in her own family, Sue set about working to help others reduce their risks. Her books bring together lowfat - low cholesterol cooking with today's lifestyles. Ranging from traditional country cuisine to modern microwave dishes these recipes and tips provide for great tasting nutrition.

Sue and her family live in Cedar Falls, Iowa. Her husband and two children have been extremly helpful with taste-testing these recipes.

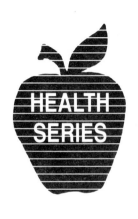

HEALTH SERIES

Fabulous Fiber Favorites
Subtitle: High Fiber Naturally

Kids Eat Healthy
Subtitle: Delicious and Nutritious

On A Healthy Wok
Subtitle: Quick and Easy

Microwave Cooking
Subtitle: Low Cholesterol and Lowfat

Healthy Entertaining
Subtitle: Here's To Your Health!

Heart Healthy Favorites
Subtitle: Low Cholesterol Cooking

Sweet & Natural
"Fruit Sweetened"

Unibook Series

1100	Cookies	2200	Beef	3700	Cajun
1200	Casseroles	2300	Holiday Collection	3800	Household Hints
1300	Meat Dishes	2400	Salads & Dressings	6100	Chinese
1400	Microwave	2500	Wild Game	6400	German
1500	Cooking for "2"	2600	Soups	6700	Italian
1600	Slow Cooking	3100	Fish & Seafood	6800	Irish
1700	Low Calorie	3200	Poultry	7000	Mexican
1900	Pastries & Pies	3300	My Own Recipes	7100	Norwegian
2000	Outdoor Grilling	3400	Low Cholesterol	7200	Swedish
2100	Appetizers	3500	Chocoholic		

TABLE OF CONTENTS

FABULOUS FIBER

A diet high in fiber is a positive, healthy diet. The presence of fiber may have a profound effect on the digestive system, and may even aid in the prevention of some noninfectious diseases. Research has indicated that a high fiber diet can have positive effects on several diseases such as: diabetes, heart disease, high blood pressure and cancer. It is suggested that an increase in dietary fiber intake will increase your overall health as well as being a positive factor in disease prevention.

A high fiber diet can easily be adopted without giving up good taste. What's more is high fiber recipes can be easy to prepare. Fiber is in, but the concept is not new. Our grandmothers called it roughage. What is new, however, is the current scientific research pointing to all of the advantages of a good healthy diet that is high in fiber.

I

Dietary fiber only comes from plants. Fiber is the part of the plant that is not digested and absorbed into the small intestine. It depends on which type of fiber is consumed as to what happens to it in the large intestine. It is important to eat foods containing both types of fiber; Soluble and insoluble fiber.

Insoluble fiber absorbs water and passes through the digestive system virtually unchanged.

Good Sources of Insoluble Fiber: (absorbs water and increases bulk)

Wheat bran
Corn bran
Dried beans
Peas
Nuts
Fruits
Vegetables

Soluble Fiber may be broken down by bacteria in the large intestine into other substances.

Good Sources of Soluble Fiber:

Beans	Apples
Peaches	Oats
Carrots	Broccoli
Citrus fruits	Barley

A high fiber diet is not only important in disease prevention, but for weight control as well. High fiber foods promote a feeling of fullness and satisfaction. Foods high in fiber tend to stay in the stomach longer, therefore keeping you from feeling hungry.

There are no recommended daily amounts for fiber, however, experts generally advise 35 to 40 grams of fiber per day for an average adult. It is important for you to consult your Doctor or diet counselor for your own personal dietary fiber needs.

It is important to slowly increase fiber rich foods, and to drink plenty of water for proper absorption.

HOW TO INCREASE YOUR DIETARY FIBER INTAKE :

1. Eat whole wheat breads instead of white breads.

2. Eat brown rice instead of white rice.

3. Switch to whole grain cereals.

4. Check labels on products for amounts of dietary fiber.

5. Eat "whole fruits" including the skin instead of just drinking juices.

6. Eat more fresh vegetables and fresh fruits.

7. Include dried beans and legumes in your diet.

8. "Slowly" increase your fiber rich food intake.

9. Increase fiber intake over a period of 3 to 4 weeks, making a few changes at a time.

10. Eat a well balanced diet.

COMMON HIGH FIBER FOODS

Almonds
Apples
Dried apricots
Artichoke
Beans
Lima beans
Blackberries
Boysenberries
Bran
Bran flakes
Whole wheat bread
Broccoli
Cabbage
Carrots
Cauliflower

Black eyed peas
Green peas
Dates
Figs
Filberts
Guavas, raw
Nuts
Bran muffins
Oatbran
Oatmeal
Parsnips
Pears, fresh
Peppers
Popcorn
Prunes, uncooked

Raspberries
Whole grain products
Rye bread
Sesame seeds
Soybeans
Squash
Strawberries
Sweet potatoes
Tomatoes
Brown rice
Sunflower seeds
Whole wheat crackers
Rye crackers
Brussels sprouts
Wheat germ
Currants

VI

The recipes in this cookbook were designed to make it easy for you to put more fiber in your diet in a healthy, natural way. Enjoy the rich taste of FABULOUS FIBER!

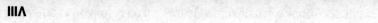

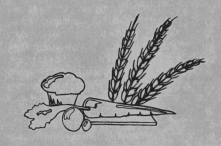

BREADS & MUFFINS

APPLE-NUT OAT BRAN MUFFINS

1 C. buttermilk
1½ C. raw oat bran
1 egg or 2 egg whites (beaten)
⅓ C. brown sugar (packed)
1 lg. cooking apple
  (cored and diced)

¼ C. chopped nuts
¼ C. raisins (optional)
2 T. corn oil or sunflower oil
1 tsp. cinnamon
½ C. whole wheat flour
1 tsp. baking soda

Combine the oat bran, buttermilk, egg, brown sugar, oil, diced apple, nuts and raisins in a medium bowl. Let stand for 10 minutes. Preheat oven to 400°. Line 12 muffin tins with paper liners. In a larger bowl, mix the wheat flour, baking soda and cinnamon. Make a well in the center and add the bran-buttermilk mixture. Stir just enough to dampen the flour; the batter should be lumpy. Do not overmix. Spoon batter into the lined muffin tins, filling each ¾ full. Bake at 400° for about 20 minutes or until golden brown and a cake tester comes out clean. The recipe can be doubled and extra muffins frozen, if desired.

1

APPLESAUCE MUFFINS

2 C. all-purpose flour
1 tsp. apple pie spice
1 tsp. baking soda
1 tsp. baking powder
⅓ C. nonfat instant dry milk

¼ tsp. salt
½ C. brown sugar
1 egg or 2 egg whites
⅓ C. vegetable oil
1¼ C. applesauce
1 C. raisins

Stir flour, spice, soda, baking powder, dry milk, salt and brown sugar together in mixer bowl at low speed for ½ minute to blend. Beat egg, oil and applesauce together to blend; add all at once to flour mixture and mix only until flour is moistened. Stir raisins or nuts into batter. Fill greased or paper-lined muffin cups about ⅔ full with batter. Bake in a preheated 400° oven for about 20 minutes or until muffins spring back when touched in the center. Makes 12.

BLUEBERRY ORANGE OATMEAL MUFFINS

1 C. quick-cooking oats
¾ C. orange juice or skim milk
1 C. all-purpose or whole wheat flour
⅓ C. sugar
1 C. fresh or frozen blueberries (thawed and drained)

1¼ tsp. baking powder
½ tsp. ground cinnamon
¼ tsp. baking soda
⅓ C. vegetable oil
2 egg whites (slightly beaten)

Heat oven to 400°. Grease bottoms only of 12 medium muffin cups or line with paper baking cups. Mix oats and orange juice in large bowl. Stir in remaining ingredients except blueberries; fold in blueberries. Divide batter evenly among muffin cups. Bake until golden brown, 18 to 22 minutes. Cool for 5 minutes and remove from pan. Makes a dozen muffins.

BLUEBERRY RAISIN BRAN MUFFINS

½ C. margarine
1 C. sugar
½ C. egg substitute
2½ C. flour
2½ tsp. baking soda
2 C. buttermilk

1 C. 100% Bran
1 C. boiling water
2 C. All Bran
½ C. chopped nuts
½ C. raisins
½ C. blueberries

Cream margarine with sugar and egg substitute. Sift flour with baking soda and add to first mixture, alternating with buttermilk; mix well. Combine 100% Bran and boiling water. Let stand for 1 minute. Add this to mixture and stir thoroughly. Then fold in All Bran, nuts, raisins and blueberries. Bake at 400° for 15 minutes. Makes 24 muffins.

BRAN APPLESAUCE PANCAKES

½ C. skim milk
½ C. egg substitute
2 T. margarine (melted)
1 C. applesauce
¾ C. 100% Bran

¾ C. all-purpose flour
2 T. granulated sugar
1 T. baking powder
¼ tsp. salt
Applesauce

In medium bowl, beat together egg substitute, skim milk, melted margarine and applesauce; stir in Bran and let set for 5 minutes. In small bowl, combine flour, sugar, baking powder and salt. Stir into bran mixture, just until moistened. For each pancake, pour or spoon a scant ¼ cup batter onto preheated, lightly greased griddle; cook, over low heat, 2 to 3 minutes or until lightly browned; turn and brown other side. Serve immediately with margarine and applesauce.

BRAN APRICOT BREAD

⅔ C. water
½ C. snipped dried apricots
½ C. raisins
¾ C. 100% Bran
1¼ C. all-purpose flour
½ C. brown sugar (firmly packed)
1 tsp. baking powder

½ tsp. baking soda
½ tsp. salt
½ C. egg substitute
¼ C. margarine (melted)
1 tsp. vanilla extract
1 (2¾ oz.) bag walnuts (chopped)

Preheat oven to 350° and grease a 9x5x3'' pan. In medium saucepan, over high heat, bring water, apricots and raisins to a boil; spoon into large bowl. Stir in 100% Bran and cool for 10 minutes. In medium bowl, combine flour, brown sugar, baking powder, baking soda and salt; set aside. With mixer on medium speed, beat egg substitute, margarine and vanilla extract into bran mixture; stir in dry ingredients; fold in walnuts. Evenly spread dough in prepared pan and bake for 50 to 55 minutes. Cool in pan for 10 minutes. Makes 1 loaf.

BRAN BAKING-POWDER BISCUITS

1 C. buttermilk
1 C. All-Bran
1½ C. all-purpose flour
½ tsp. baking soda

1 T. sugar
2 tsp. baking powder
½ tsp. salt
⅓ C. shortening

Mix milk and bran; stir to mix well and let stand until needed. Stir flour, soda, sugar, baking powder and salt together to blend. Cut shortening into flour mixture until it resembles a coarse meal; add bran and milk mixture and stir with a fork to form a soft dough. Turn onto a floured surface and knead lightly about 10 times. Pat dough to about ¾" thickness. Cut dough with a floured 2" round cutter. Place biscuits on a lightly greased baking sheet. Bake in a preheated 400° oven for 15 to 20 minutes or until lightly browned. Serve warm.

BRAN PANCAKES

1 C. Bran Buds
2 C. skim milk
2 C. all-purpose flour
1 tsp. salt

1 tsp. baking powder
1 tsp. baking soda
⅓ C. light molasses
¼ C. vegetable oil
2 lg. eggs or 4 egg whites

Stir bran into milk and set aside for at least 5 minutes. Stir flour, salt, baking powder and soda together to blend. Beat molasses, oil and eggs into bran mixture; add to flour mixture and stir until smooth. Pour about ⅓ cup batter onto a lightly greased preheated 375° griddle. Cook about 3 minutes or until bubbles form on the surface and the edge of the pancake is dry; turn and cook 2 minutes longer until nicely browned. Repeat with remaining batter.

BRAN-CRAN BREAD

2 C. whole cranberries
1½ C. oat-bran cereal
1 tsp. grated orange peel
¾ C. granulated sugar
⅓ C. brown sugar
½ C. chopped walnuts

2½ C. all-purpose flour
3 tsp. baking powder
½ tsp. ground allspice
¼ C. vegetable oil
1 container egg substitute

Chop the cranberries and add to the oat-bran cereal along with the orange peel and sugars. Mix together the flour, baking powder and allspice. Add the oil and egg substitute. Blend in the cranberry mixture and walnuts. Spray 3-6x3" loaf pans with vegetable oil cooking spray and divide the batter between the pans. Bake for 40 to 50 minutes at 350° or until a toothpick comes out clean.

CARROT OATMEAL MUFFINS

1 C. flour
2 tsp. baking powder
½ tsp. soda
¼ tsp. salt
½ tsp. cinnamon
½ C. brown sugar (packed)

1 C. milk
1 egg (beaten) or
    2 egg whites
¼ C. melted margarine
1 C. shredded carrots
1 C. quick-cooking oats

In a large mixing bowl, blend together the flour, baking powder, soda, salt and cinnamon. Add the brown sugar, milk, egg and margarine. Mix thoroughly. Add the carrots and oats; mix well. Spoon the batter into greased muffin pan cups, filling them ⅔ full. Bake at 375° for 25 minutes. Serve hot or cold. Makes 1 dozen.

CARROT-RAISIN MUFFINS

2¼ C. flour
¾ C. wheat germ
1 T. baking powder
1½ tsp. cinnamon
1 tsp. salt
¾ C. raisins

½ tsp. baking soda
½ C. egg substitute
1 C. sugar
½ C. vegetable oil
½ C. milk
2 C. carrots, shredded
(about 4 carrots)

Combine flour, wheat germ, baking powder, cinnamon, salt and baking soda; set aside. Beat egg substitute, sugar and oil together in small bowl. Gradually add egg mixture alternating with milk to flour mixture. Stir in carrots and raisins. Fill muffin tins or paper cups ⅔ full and bake at 350° for 20 minutes or until wooden toothpick inserted in center comes out clean. Serve hot or freeze and reheat in microwave oven.

CEREAL WHOLE-WHEAT MUFFINS

1½ C. uncooked Quaker
  Whole-Wheat cereal
1 C. all-purpose flour
1 T. baking powder
⅓ C. sugar

¼ tsp. salt
1 C. skim milk
1 egg or 2 egg whites
¼ C. vegetable oil

Place uncooked cereal, flour, baking powder, sugar and salt in mixer bowl; mix 1 minute at low speed or until well blended. Mix milk, egg and oil together until smooth; add to flour mixture and beat at low speed only until flour is moistened. Fill greased or paper-lined muffin tins about ⅔ full with batter. Bake in a preheated 400° oven for about 20 minutes or until done. Makes 12 muffins.

CORN BREAD

¾ C. cornmeal
1 C. flour
3 tsp. baking powder
¼ tsp. salt

¼ C. molasses
¾ C. skim milk
¼ C. egg substitute (beaten)
2 T. safflower oil

Sift together dry ingredients; add remaining ingredients. Mix with a spoon. Bake in a 9" round pan at 375° for 30 minutes.

EASY BRAN BISCUITS

2 C. biscuit mix
1 T. sugar
½ tsp. baking powder
½ C. Bran Buds

Amount of liquid specified on
  biscuit mix package
2 T. water

Stir biscuit mix, sugar and baking powder together in a bowl. Combine bran, specified liquid and water; let stand 5 minutes and add to biscuit mix. Mix lightly with a fork until flour is moistened. Knead dough several times in the bowl; turn out onto a lightly floured surface. Pat dough out to between ½ and ¾" thickness; cut into biscuits. Place biscuits on greased baking sheet. Bake in a preheated 425° oven for about 20 minutes or until biscuits are lightly browned. Makes 8 to 10 biscuits.

GOOD MORNING MUFFINS

2¼ C. oat-bran cereal
¼ C. chopped nuts
   (walnuts, pecans, or peanuts)
¼ C. raisins (or dates or
   currants)
1 T. baking powder
2 T. vegetable oil

¼ C. brown sugar
   (or honey or molasses)
1¼ C. skim milk or
   evaporated skim milk
2 egg whites or
   ½ C. egg substitute

Combine oat-bran cereal, nuts, raisins and baking powder. Stir in the brown sugar. Mix milk, egg whites and oil together; blend in with the oat-bran mixture. Line muffin pans with paper baking cups and fill with batter. Bake at 425° for 15 to 17 minutes. Test for doneness with a toothpick. It should come out moist. Makes 12 muffins.

HONEY RAISIN BRAN MUFFINS

1¼ C. all-purpose flour
1 T. baking powder
¼ tsp. salt
2½ C. raisin bran cereal

1 C. skim milk
⅓ C. honey
2 egg whites
3 T. vegetable oil

Sift together flour, baking powder and salt; set aside. In a large mixing bowl, stir together raisin bran cereal, milk and honey. Let stand for 1 or 2 minutes or until cereal is softened. Add egg whites and oil, beat well. Add flour mixture, stirring only until combined. Divide batter evenly into 12 greased 2½" muffin pan cups. Bake at 400° for 18 to 20 minutes or until lightly browned.

HEALTHFUL OATMEAL BREAD

¾ C. boiling water
½ C. old-fashioned rolled
  oats
3 T. margarine
¼ C. honey
1 tsp. salt
1 env. active dry yeast
¼ C. very warm water

½ tsp. sugar
¼ container egg substitute
  (equal to 1 egg)
2 C. all-purpose flour
¾ C. oat-bran cereal
  (milled to flour in blender)

Stir together the boiling water, rolled oats, margarine, honey and salt in a large bowl until well mixed. Let cool to warm. Sprinkle the packet of yeast over the very warm water in a 1-cup container; add the ½ teaspoon sugar. Stir to dissolve the yeast and let it stand for about 10 minutes or until the mixture bubbles. Next add the yeast mixture, egg substitute, 1½ cups all-purpose flour and the oat bran to the oatmeal mixture. Beat with an electric mixer at low speed for 2 minutes while gradually adding the rest of the flour. Put the dough into a 9x5x3'' loaf pan sprayed with vegetable oil spray. Cover with waxed paper and a towel and place the pan in a warm place away from drafts. Let the dough double in bulk, about 45 minutes. Bake in a preheated oven at 375° for about 1 hour. Remove the bread from the pan and let it cool.

HONEY-WHOLE WHEAT BUTTER HORNS

¾ C. milk
⅓ C. honey
2 T. sorghum
½ C. white sugar
2¼ tsp. salt
6 T. margarine

¾ C. warm water
3 pkgs. dry yeast
¾ C. egg substitute
3 C. stone-ground whole
  wheat flour
3¾ C. enriched white flour
¾ C. wheat germ

Scald milk and add honey, sorghum, sugar, salt and margarine. Pour into large mixing bowl to cool. Soften yeast in warm water. Add 2 cups whole wheat flour and 1 cup white flour to milk mixture and beat well. Add egg substitute and mix well. Add softened yeast and mix well. Add wheat germ and remaining flour, reserving ½ cup white flour to kneading and rolling; mix well. Turn out on lightly floured board, cover and let rest for 5 minutes. Knead until smooth. Place into large greased bowl and let rise in warm place until doubled in bulk. Punch down and divide into 3 equal portions. Roll on lightly floured board into circular shape approximately ½" thick. Spread with melted margarine. Cut into 12 pie-shaped pieces and roll, starting with the wide end. Put each dozen on greased baking sheet (approximately 14x16"), curving slightly and let rise until light. Bake at 350° for 7 to 10 minutes or until done and lightly golden brown. Makes 3 dozen.

MOLASSES MUFFINS WITH BRAN

2½ C. oat-bran cereal
1 T. baking powder
¼ C. raisins
¼ C. chopped nuts

1¼ C. skim milk
2 T. vegetable oil
2 egg whites
¼ C. molasses

Blend dry ingredients in a bowl. Mix all other ingredients in a blender and add to the dry ingredients. Stir to mix. Line the muffin pan with paper baking cups and fill with the batter. Bake at 425° for 16 minutes.

MOLASSES MUFFINS WITH WHEAT GERM

2 C. all-purpose flour
1 C. wheat germ
1 T. baking powder
1 egg or 2 egg whites

¾ C. skim milk
¼ C. vegetable oil
¼ C. molasses
¼ C. light brown sugar

Place flour, wheat germ and baking powder in mixer bowl; mix at low speed for 1 minute or until well blended. Combine egg, milk, oil, molasses and brown sugar; beat together until well blended. Add all at once to flour mixture and mix at low speed only until flour is moistened. Fill paper-lined muffin tins about ⅔ full. Bake in a preheated 375° oven for 20 to 25 minutes or until golden. Makes 12 muffins.

NUTRITIOUS MUFFINS

1 C. enriched white flour
½ C. whole wheat flour
½ C. oatmeal
2 tsp. baking soda
1 C. raisins
Dash salt

½ C. wheat germ
¼ C. egg substitute
½ C. safflower oil
1 C. skim milk
¼ C. honey

Combine flours, oatmeal, baking soda, salt, wheat germ, raisins and egg substitute. In another bowl mix oil, milk and honey; add to flour mixture; blend. Pour into paper-lined muffin cups. Bake at 400° for 25 minutes.

OATMEAL BUNS

⅓ C. oil or margarine
1 tsp. salt
⅓ C. brown sugar
1 C. oatmeal (not instant)
1¼ C. boiling water

1 pkg. dry yeast, dissolved in
 ¼ C. warm water
1 egg (beaten) or
 2 egg whites
4 C. flour

Pour the boiling water over the oil, salt, brown sugar and oatmeal. Let stand until lukewarm. Dissolve the yeast in the warm water and add to lukewarm oatmeal mixture. Add the beaten egg and 2 cups flour; mix well. Add 2 more cups of flour and mix. Let rise until double. Shape into buns and place on sprayed round cake pans. Let rise until doubled. Bake at 375° for 12 minutes or until light brown on top.

PEANUT BUTTER MUFFINS

2 C. all-purpose flour
1 T. baking powder
1 tsp. salt
½ C. sugar

¾ C. crunchy peanut butter
2 eggs or
  ½ C. egg substitute
⅓ C. vegetable oil
1 C. milk

Place flour, baking powder, salt and sugar together in mixer bowl; mix at low speed ½ minute or until well blended. Add peanut butter and mix about 1 minute at low speed or until peanut butter is cut into small pieces throughout the flour. Mix eggs, oil and milk together until well blended; add to flour mixture and mix only until flour is moistened. Fill greased or paper-lined muffin tins about ⅔ full with batter. Bake in a preheated 400° oven for about 20 minutes or until done.

PEAR MUFFINS

2¼ C. oat-bran cereal
3 T. brown sugar
1 T. baking powder
½ tsp. cinnamon
¼ tsp. vanilla

2 egg whites
2 T. vegetable oil
¾ C. skim milk
1 lg. ripe pear or 2 sm. pears
   (peeled and cored)

Blend dry ingredients in a large bowl. Mix all the other ingredients, including the pear, in a blender at low speed. Combine with the dry ingredients and mix. Fill baking cups with batter. Bake at 425° for 17 minutes.

PINEAPPLE BRAN MUFFIN

2¼ C. oat-bran cereal
¼ C. brown sugar
1 T. baking powder
½ C. skim milk

2-8 oz. cans crushed
   pineapple in its own juice
   (unsweetened)
2 egg whites
2 T. vegetable oil

Blend dry ingredients in a large bowl. Mix the milk, 1 can crushed pineapple with juice, egg whites and oil in a bowl or blender. Combine the ingredients and mix. Drain the second can of pineapple and add to the mixture. Fill muffin cups with batter. Bake at 425° for 17 minutes.

PINEAPPLE PUMPKIN MUFFINS

2¼ C. oat-bran cereal
3 T. brown sugar
1 T. baking powder
½ tsp. nutmeg
½ tsp. cinnamon
¼ C. raisins

½ C. canned pumpkin
½ C. frozen pineapple-juice
  concentrate
¾ C. skim milk
2 T. vegetable oil
2 egg whites

Blend dry ingredients in a large bowl. Put all other ingredients in a blender. Mix with the dry ingredients and stir just to mix. Fill muffin cups with batter and bake at 425° for 17 minutes.

PINEAPPLE-CARROT BREAD

1-8 oz. can crushed pineapple
  (undrained)
¾ C. egg substitute
½ C. margarine (melted)
¾ C. 100% Bran
1¾ C. all-purpose flour
¾ C. sugar

1 T. low-sodium baking
  powder
1 tsp. baking soda
1 tsp. ground cinnamon
½ tsp. ground nutmeg
1 C. shredded carrots
½ C. chopped dates

Drain pineapple, reserving juice; add water to make ½ cup liquid. In large bowl, beat together, pineapple juice, egg substitute and margarine until well blended. Stir in 100% Bran; let stand for 5 minutes. In small bowl, stir together flour, sugar, baking powder, baking soda, cinnamon and nutmeg. Stir into bran mixture. Stir in carrots, dates and pineapple. Spread in greased and floured 9x5x3" loaf pan. Bake at 350° for 50 to 60 minutes or until toothpick inserted in center comes out clean. Cool in pan on wire rack for 10 minutes. Remove from pan; cool completely on wire rack. 30

RAISIN-ZUCCHINI BREAD

¾ C. egg substitute (beaten)
1 C. safflower oil
2 C. sugar
2 C. grated zucchini
3 tsp. vanilla
3 C. all-purpose flour
½ tsp. salt
1 tsp. soda
3 tsp. cinnamon
½ tsp. baking powder
1 C. raisins
Tub safflower margarine

Combine egg substitute, oil, sugar, zucchini and vanilla. In another bowl, combine remaining ingredients, except raisins. Gradually add to zucchini mixture; blend and stir in raisins. Pour into 2 loaf pans that have been greased with margarine. Bake at 350° for 1 hour. Makes 2 loaves.

RASPBERRY BRAN MUFFINS

1 C. fresh or frozen raspberries
1 C. all-purpose flour
1 C. unprocessed oat bran
¼ C. sugar
3 tsp. baking powder

¼ tsp. salt
2 egg whites
1 C. milk
¼ C. cooking oil

Partially thaw frozen raspberries. Do not completely thaw. In bowl stir together flour, bran, sugar, baking powder and salt. Make a well in center. In a small bowl, combine egg whites, milk and oil; add all at once to flour mixture. Stir just until moistened. Fold in raspberries. Grease bottoms of muffin cups or line with paper bake cups. Fill ⅔ full. Bake in 400° oven for about 20 minutes or until done. Remove from pan. Cool slightly on wire racks. Makes 12.

RYE MUFFINS

1 C. all-purpose flour	⅓ C. nonfat instant dry milk
1 C. rye flour	1 T. caraway seed
4 tsp. baking powder	1 C. water
½ tsp. salt	⅓ C. vegetable oil
⅓ C. brown sugar	1 egg or 2 egg whites

Place flours, baking powder, salt, brown sugar, dry milk and caraway seed in mixer bowl; mix at low speed for 1 minute to blend. Mix water, oil and egg together until well blended; add to flour mixture. Beat at low speed only until flour is moistened. Fill buttered or paper-lined muffin tins about ½ full with batter. Bake in a preheated 400° oven for 20 to 25 minutes or until muffins spring back when touched in the center. Makes 12.

STRAWBERRY BRAN MUFFINS

2¼ C. oat-bran cereal
¼ C. brown sugar
1 T. baking powder
½ C. skim milk
¾ C. canned strawberry
  nectar or strawberry juice

¾ C. fresh or frozen
  strawberries
2 egg whites
2 T. vegetable oil

Blend dry ingredients in a bowl. Mix the milk, strawberry nectar, strawberries, egg whites and oil in a bowl or blender. (Save 12 pieces of fresh strawberry to place on top of the muffins.) Combine with the dry ingredients and mix. Line muffin cups with paper baking cups and fill with batter. Arrange a piece of strawberry on each. Bake at 425° for 17 minutes.

WHOLE-WHEAT BISCUITS

1 C. whole-wheat flour
1 C. all-purpose flour
1 T. baking powder
1 T. brown sugar

½ tsp. salt
⅓ C. shortening
1 C. buttermilk

Combine flours, baking powder, brown sugar and salt together to mix. Cut shortening into flour mixture until it resembles a coarse meal; add buttermilk and stir with a fork to form a soft dough. Knead several times on a lightly floured surface and roll dough to about ¾" thickness. Cut into biscuits. Place biscuits on a greased baking sheet. Bake in a preheated 400° oven for 15 to 20 minutes or until lightly browned.

YOGURT-CARROT SQUARES

2 C. whole-wheat flour
½ C. all-purpose flour
2 tsp. baking soda
1 tsp. baking powder
1 tsp. salt
1 tsp. grated lemon peel

1-8 oz. carton lowfat
  plain yogurt
1 C. finely grated carrots
½ C. molasses
½ C. chopped nuts
1 egg or 2 egg whites

Combine flours, soda, baking powder, salt and lemon peel in mixer bowl; mix at low speed for 1 minute or until well blended. Combine yogurt, carrots, molasses, nuts and egg; mix to blend. Add to flour mixture and beat at low speed only until flour is moistened. Spread batter in a greased 9" square pan. Bake in a preheated 350° oven for 25 to 30 minutes or until sides pull away from the pan.

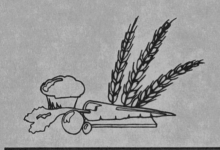

MAIN DISHES

BARBECUE BURGERS

1 egg or 2 egg whites
1 tsp. onion powder
1 tsp. prepared horseradish
1 tsp. Worcestershire sauce
¼ tsp. salt
½ tsp. chili powder

1 T. barbecue sauce
1 C. Wheat Chex,
 crushed to ½ C.
1 lb. lean ground beef
Barbecue sauce

Combine egg, onion powder, horseradish, Worcestershire sauce, salt, chili powder and barbecue sauce; mix to blend. Add Wheat Chex and beef and mix lightly to blend. Shape into 4 equal patties about 1'' thick. Broil or grill 16 to 18 minutes or until done; brush with barbecue sauce during cooking. Makes 4 patties.

BEEF AND GREEN BEANS

8 oz. semi-frozen lean round
  or sirloin steak, cut 1" thick
2 T. low sodium soy sauce
1 tsp. sugar
1 T. cornstarch
¾ tsp. garlic salt

1 T. sherry
2 T. vegetable oil
1 lb. frozen green beans
Cooked rice

Cut beef, with a very sharp knife, diagonally across the grain into very thin slices. Combine soy sauce, sugar, cornstarch, garlic salt and sherry; dredge beef in mixture. Heat oil in a heavy frying pan. Add meat to oil and cook and stir over moderate heat until meat is browned. Add drained canned green beans plus ¼ cup liquid or frozen green beans. Cover and simmer, stirring occasionally, until canned beans are hot or frozen beans are tender crisp. Serve hot over rice.

CHICKEN PARISIENNE

2 pkgs. frozen broccoli
2 T. special margarine
2 T. flour
¼ tsp. white pepper
2 C. chicken broth

½ C. skim milk
1½ T. grated
  Parmesan cheese
18 thin slices cooked chicken

Undercook broccoli 2 minutes less than package suggests; drain and spread on bottom of a baking dish. Melt the margarine in a saucepan; blend in the flour and pepper. Add the broth and milk, stirring steadily to the boiling point. Cook over low heat 5 minutes. Mix in the cheese. Pour half the sauce over the broccoli. Arrange the chicken over it and cover with the remaining sauce. Bake in a 425° oven for 10 minutes.

BETTER BURGERS

1 slightly beaten egg white
⅓ C. bulgur
¼ C. catsup
1 T. snipped fresh parsley
1 tsp. dried Italian seasoning
  (crushed)
¼ tsp. garlic salt

⅛ tsp. pepper
1 lb. lean ground beef
4 whole wheat hamburger
  buns (split and toasted)
Lettuce leaves
4 tomato slices
Alfalfa sprouts (optional)

In a medium mixing bowl combine egg white, bulgur, catsup, parsley, Italian seasoning, garlic salt and pepper. Add ground beef and mix well. Shape mixture into four ½" thick patties. Grill patties on an uncovered grill directly over medium-hot coals for 12 to 15 minutes or to desired doneness, turning once. (Or, place patties on unheated rack of a broiler pan. Broil 3" from heat for 10 to 12 minutes or to desired doneness, turning once.) Serve patties on toasted wheat hamburger buns with lettuce, tomato slices and alfalfa sprouts, if desired.

For Microwave: Prepare and shape patties as directed. Arrange in an 8x8x2" microwave-safe baking dish. Cover with waxed paper. Microcook on 100% power (HIGH) for 5 to 7 minutes or to desired doneness, giving dish a half-turn and turning patties over once. Serve as directed.

CHICKEN PRIMAVERA

1 carrot, cut crosswise in
   ¼" slices
½ green bell pepper, cut
   in ¼" strips
4 oz. mushrooms, quartered
1 broccoli stalk, broken in
   flowerets, stem cut
   crosswise in ¼" slices
2 T. margarine
5 green onion, thinly
   sliced
1 lb. boneless skinned
   chicken breasts, cut in ¼" strips

2 T. all-purpose flour
1½ C. chicken broth
1 C. dry white wine
1½ tsp. dried leaf basil
Dash hot-pepper sauce
1 tomato, cut in 8 wedges
2 C. multi-colored rotini
   (6 oz.), cooked, drained
Salt (optional)
Freshly ground pepper

In a large saucepan, steam carrot, bell pepper, mushrooms and broccoli over boiling water 5 minutes or until crisp-tender. Remove from pan; set aside. In a medium-size deep skillet, melt margarine over medium heat. Add onion; saute until softened. Add chicken; saute, stirring constantly, 3 to 4 minutes or until chicken is no longer pink. Using a slotted spoon, remove onion and chicken; set aside. Stir flour into fat remaining in pan; cook about 2 minutes or until bubbly. Stir in broth, wine, basil and hot-pepper sauce. Cook, stirring continuously, until thickened. Stir in tomato, steamed vegetables and chicken mixture. Pour over rotini; toss to combine. Season with salt and pepper. Serve hot. Makes 4 servings.

CHICKEN WITH NUT GRAVY

2 (2½ lb. ea.) broilers (cut-up)	1 C. chopped onions
½ C. flour	1½ C. diced green peppers
½ tsp. salt	2 tsp. tomato paste
4 T. special oil	2 C. chicken broth
3 T. cognac	¼ C. chopped walnuts

Dip chicken in a mixture of the flour and salt. Heat 3 tablespoons oil in a skillet; brown the chicken pieces in it well. Transfer to a casserole. Heat the cognac, pour it over the chicken and set aflame. Add the remaining oil to the skillet; saute the onions and green peppers 10 minutes. Blend in the tomato paste, broth and walnuts. Cover and bake in 350° oven for 45 minutes or until tender. Remove cover for last 10 minutes.

CHICKEN-SQUASH BAKE

1 T. olive oil
1 lg. garlic clove, minced
12 oz. cooked chicken, cut in
  1" pieces (about 3 C.)
4 oz. mushrooms, sliced
3 C. cooked spaghetti squash
1 (10 oz.) pkg. frozen green
  peas, thawed

2½ T. grated
  Parmesan cheese
1 tsp. ground leaf thyme
1½ C. low sodium
  tomato sauce
Freshly ground pepper

Preheat oven to 400°. Grease a shallow 3-quart casserole dish. In a small skillet, heat olive oil over medium heat. Add garlic; cook until garlic starts to brown. In a medium-size bowl, toss garlic, chicken, mushrooms, squash, peas, cheese and thyme until combined. Add tomato sauce. Season with salt and pepper. Toss to combine. Pour mixture into greased dish. Bake uncovered, in preheated oven about 25 minutes or until hot. Makes 4 servings.

CURRIED CHICKEN

½ C. chopped onion
2 C. chicken broth
2 C. skim milk
½ C. flour
¼ tsp. salt
1 T. curry powder
¼ tsp. ground ginger
1 T. lemon juice
4 C. cooked chicken (diced)

1 (8 oz.) can sliced water
   chestnuts
Steamed rice
Peanuts for garnish (optional)
Raisins for garnish (optional)
Pineapple chunks for garnish
   (optional)
Homemade chutney
   (optional)

In small amount of chicken broth, saute onion until tender; add remaining broth. Bring to a boil. Shake milk and flour in a covered container to form a smooth paste; gradually add to boiling broth, stirring constantly until thick. Add seasonings. Pour lemon juice over chicken; add to sauce. Stir in water chestnuts. Heat. Serve over steamed rice. May garnish with unsalted peanuts, raisins, pineapple chunks and chutney.

LEMON HERB GRILLED CHICKEN WITH VEGETABLE KEBABS

2 to 2½ lbs. chicken pieces
¾ C. vegetable oil
¾ C. lemon juice
2 tsp. seasoned salt
2 tsp. paprika
2 tsp. sweet basil
2 tsp. thyme
½ tsp. garlic powder
Zucchini, mushroom,
  peppers, tomatoes

Place chicken in heavy plastic bag. Combine remaining ingredients except vegetables; pour over chicken. Seal bag. Marinate* in refrigerator several hours or overnight. Make vegetable kebabs by threading 1" chunks of vegetables on skewers. Broil or grill chicken and vegetables 4" from heat source 5 to 8 minutes per side for vegetables and 15 to 20 minutes per side for chicken or until done. Baste often with marinade.

*(To shorten marinating time, place chicken and marinade mixture in 8x12" baking dish. Microwave, covered, on HIGH 10 minutes. Grill 8 to 10 minutes per side.)

RICE-VEGETABLE-MEAT CASSEROLE

1 lb. lean hamburger
1 T. oil
2 C. sliced potatoes
½ C. sliced onion

1 C. sliced carrots
½ C. raw white rice
2 C. tomatoes
Salt and pepper, to taste

Brown hamburger in oil, crumbing it with a fork and season to taste. Place in 2-quart casserole in layers, first meat, then sprinkle rice, next onion, carrots, potatoes and last, tomatoes. Season each layer lightly. Add just enough hot water or tomato juice to just show through. Cover casserole and bake at 325° for 2 hours.

STUFFED PEPPERS WITH CHICKEN

4 med. green peppers
½ C. chopped onion
1 (1 lb.) can stewed tomatoes
2 C. cooked barley or rice
¼ tsp. Tabasco sauce

Dash pepper
3 cooked chicken breasts
  (deboned and cubed)
¾ C. grated lowfat
  mozzarella or
  lowfat Cheddar cheese

Remove tops of green peppers; remove seeds and membrane. Saute onion in small amount of tomato liquid; add tomatoes, rice or barley, Tabasco, pepper, chicken and ½ of the cheese. Stand peppers upright in an 8" square baking dish; stuff with tomato-barley filling. Bake uncovered at 350° for 25 to 30 minutes. Sprinkle with remaining cheese. Return to oven until cheese melts.

TURKEY AND SAUERKRAUT

1 (1 lb.) can sauerkraut,
  drained, rinsed
½ sm. head green cabbage,
  finely shredded
½ med. onion, chopped
1 lg. Granny Smith apple,
  chopped
1 lg. garlic clove, minced

2 tsp. juniper berries, crushed
1 bay leaf
11 sm. new red potatoes
2 (1-lb.) turkey thighs,
  skinned
3 C. beer

In a Dutch oven,, combine sauerkraut, cabbage, onion, apple, garlic, juniper berries and bay leaf. Place potatoes and turkey over cabbage mixture. Add beer. Bring to a boil over medium heat. Reduce heat, cover and simmer 45 minutes or until turkey and potatoes are tender. Discard bay leaf. Cut turkey in serving pieces. Makes 6 servings. Serve with rye bread, if desired.

TURKEY MEATBALLS

¼ C. oat-bran cereal
¼ tsp. oregano
¼ tsp. black pepper
¼ tsp. thyme
½ T. grated Parmesan cheese

1 lg. garlic clove
 (finely minced)
¼ C. chopped onion
¼ C. chopped green pepper
1 lb. ground turkey breast

Blend dry ingredients in a bowl. Add all the remaining ingredients, except turkey. Then mix in the ground turkey and form into 12 to 16 balls. Spray a nonstick pan with nonstick coating. Fry turkey balls, uncovered until browned. Serve over spaghetti and meatless tomato sauce. Makes about 14 meatballs.

TURKEY MEATBALLS IN PAPRIKA SAUCE

1 lb. ground turkey breast
¼ C. oat-bran cereal
1 T. ketchup
¼ tsp. black pepper
1 garlic clove (finely minced)
1 T. paprika

1 C. chicken bouillon
1½ C. finely sliced onions
½ C. skim milk
¼ C. flour
2 T. minced parsley

Blend the turkey, oat bran, ketchup, pepper and garlic. Mold into small balls. Fry in a nonstick pan sprayed with Pam. Remove the balls when browned. Add the chicken bouillon to the pan along with the sliced onions. Bring to a boil and simmer until the onions are tender. In another bowl, slowly blend the skim milk into the G cup flour until smooth. Then slowly drizzle in the chicken bouillon and onions; blend. Cook over medium heat, stirring until thick. Add paprika to the finished sauce. Pour over the meatballs. Garnish with parsley. Serve with mashed potatoes. Use skim milk and Butter Buds for the potatoes.

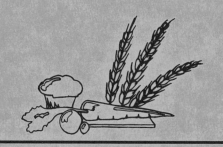

MICROWAVE

APRICOT BRAN BREAD

1 C. all-purpose flour
1 C. oat bran cereal
½ tsp. baking soda
1 tsp. baking powder
¼ tsp. salt (optional)
½ C. brown sugar

2½ oz. chopped walnuts
½ C. egg substitute
¼ C. vegetable oil
1 tsp. vanilla
½ C. snipped dried apricots
½ C. raisins
½ C. skim milk

Combine the first 6 items; set dry ingredients aside. In a large mixing bowl, blend the egg substitutes, oil, vanilla and milk; add the dry ingredients and mix until moistened. Fold in dried fruit and walnuts. Pour into a 9" microwave-safe tube pan coated lightly with vegetable oil cooking spray. Microwave on MEDIUM (50% power) for 6 to 8 minutes. Rotate pan ½ turn and continue on HIGH (100% power) for 5 to 6 minutes. The cake will be moist to touch. Allow cake to stand 5 minutes. Makes 8 servings. 53

BRAN MUFFINS

⅓ C. water
⅔ C. whole bran cereal
1¼ C. all-purpose flour
⅓ C. granulated sugar
2 tsp. baking powder
¼ tsp. salt
¾ tsp. pumpkin pie spice
2 egg whites, beaten
⅓ C. skim milk

⅓ C. safflower oil
1 sm. apple, cored and finely chopped
¼ C. chopped walnuts
2 T. chopped pecans
2 T. all-purpose flour
1 T. brown sugar
1 T. safflower oil

In a glass measure, microwave the water on HIGH (100% power) for 1 to 1½ minutes or until boiling. Place cereal in a small bowl and add water; let stand 10 minutes. Meanwhile, in a large bowl, combine the flour, granulated sugar, baking powder, salt and pie spice; mix well. Stir egg whites, milk and oil into the cereal mixture; add to the dry ingredients, stirring just until moistened. Fold in apple and walnuts. Fill microwave-safe cupcake dish, which has been lined with paper baking cups, ⅔ full. Combine the 2 tablespoons pecans, flour, brown sugar and oil. Sprinkle atop muffins. Microwave, uncovered on HIGH for 2½ to 3 minutes for 6 muffins, rotating dish every minute. Wooden pick inserted in center should come out clean when muffins are done. Remove muffins from dish and let stand 5 to 10 minutes before serving. Makes 12 muffins

BRAN PEANUT BUTTER COOKIES

¾ C. peanut butter
½ C. margarine
¾ C. brown sugar (firmly packed)
½ C. egg substitute
¾ tsp. vanilla

1 C. flour
1 C. bran cereal
¼ C. quick oats
½ tsp. baking soda
¼ tsp. salt

In mixer bowl, combine the peanut butter, margarine, brown sugar, egg substitute and vanilla; with mixer, cream until light and fluffy. Combine flour, bran, oats, baking soda and salt; mix well. Blend flour mixture into creamed mixture. Drop 5 to 8 rounded teaspoonfuls in large ring on wax paper, place on bottom of microwave-safe plate. Drop 1 or 2 in center. Microwave on MEDIUM (50% power) for 1 to 4 minutes or until just dry on surface. Turn plate ¼ turn after first 45 seconds, then every 20 seconds until cookies are done. Makes 2 to 2½ dozen.

BRAN RAISIN MUFFINS

1 ½ C. all-purpose flour
2 C. bran cereal
¾ C. sugar
¾ C. raisins
5 tsp. baking powder

1 ½ tsp. salt
½ tsp. cinnamon
1 ½ C. skim milk
½ C. egg substitute
½ C. safflower oil
¼ C. chopped nuts

In a large bowl, combine the flour, bran cereal, sugar, raisins, baking powder, salt and cinnamon; mix well. In a glass measure, mix the milk, egg substitute and oil. Add liquid all at once to dry ingredients, stirring just till moistened. Spoon batter into paper-lined microwave-safe muffin cups. Sprinkle muffins with chopped nuts. Microwave on medium-high (70% power) 6 muffins at a time for 2½ to 4 minutes turning and checking muffins after 2 minutes. Check often, wooden picks inserted in center should come out clean when muffins are done. Makes 24 muffins.

CARROT-DATE BREAD

1 C. all-purpose flour
¾ C. granulated sugar
1 tsp. baking powder
1 tsp. baking soda
¾ tsp. salt
½ tsp. ground cinnamon

¼ tsp. ground nutmeg
½ C. safflower oil
½ C. egg substitute
½ C. chopped dates
1½ C. shredded carrots

In a large bowl, combine the flour, sugar, baking powder, baking soda, salt, cinnamon and nutmeg; mix well. Add the oil, egg substitute, dates and carrots. Beat at medium speed for 1 minute. Spread batter in a 9x5" microwave-safe loaf pan lined on the bottom with wax paper. Shield ends of loaf pan with 2" wide strips of foil, covering 1" of batter. Place loaf on an inverted microwave-safe saucer. Microwave on MEDIUM (50% power) for 9 minutes, rotating dish ¼ turn every 3 minutes. Remove foil. Microwave on HIGH (100% power) for 2 to 5 minutes, checking often for doneness. Wooden pick inserted in center will come out clean when done. Let stand 5 to 10 minutes before removing. Loosen edges and turn out on rack. Remove wax paper and cool completely before cutting.

DATE OATMEAL BARS

1 ¼ C. quick cooking oats
1 ¼ C. all-purpose flour
½ tsp. baking soda
⅛ tsp. salt
1 tsp. vanilla

½ C. brown sugar
¼ C. margarine
½ C. pitted dates
¼ C. water
2 ½ T. sugar
½ T. lemon juice

Mix the first 7 ingredients until crumbly in texture. Divide oatmeal mixture into 2 portions. Spread half of the mixture evenly over the bottom on 8x8x2" microwave-safe dish coated with vegetable oil cooking spray. Place dish on an inverted saucer in microwave. Microwave on MEDIUM (50% power) for 5 to 10 minutes or until just done, rotating every 2 minutes. Combine dates, water, sugar and lemon juice in a glass mixing bowl. Microwave on HIGH (100% power) 3 to 5 minutes or until thick and smooth, stirring every minute. Spread date mixture over cooled oatmeal mixture. Spread remaining half of oatmeal mixture over the filling and pat down so that the top is smooth and even. Microwave on HIGH 8 to 10 minutes or until crumbly mixture is cooked; rotating ½ turn every 2 minutes. Top should be moist. Cut into bars while still warm.

CHICKEN-ASPARAGUS PITAS

¼ C. cold water
2 T. soy sauce (low-salt)
5 tsp. cornstarch
1 tsp. vinegar
½ tsp. dry mustard
½ tsp. ground ginger

1-10 oz. pkg. frozen cup
  asparagus
¼ C. chopped canned water
  chestnuts
¼ C. sliced green onion
1½ C. chopped cooked lean,
  white chicken
2 lg. pita bread rounds

In a 1½-quart microwave-safe casserole, combine water, soy sauce, cornstarch, vinegar, mustard and ginger. If necessary, break up the frozen block of asparagus. Stir asparagus, water chestnuts and green onion into sauce mixture. Microwave, uncovered, on HIGH (100% power) about 5 minutes or until asparagus is crisp-tender, stirring every 2 minutes. Stir in cooked chicken. Cook, uncovered, on HIGH for 3 to 4 minutes or until chicken is heated through. Cut pita breads in half crosswise. Spoon the chicken-asparagus mixture into the pita halves. Makes 4 servings.

FRESH RASPBERRY CRISP

1 qt. fresh raspberries
2 T. granulated sugar
¼ C. margarine

⅓ C. flour
⅓ C. packed brown sugar
¾ C. rolled oats

Place raspberries in bottom of a 9" square microwave-safe cake pan. Sprinkle with granulated sugar. Blend margarine, flour, brown sugar and oats until mixture resembles coarse meal. Sprinkle the oat mixture over the raspberries. Microwave on MEDIUM (50% power) for 5 to 10 minutes. Let stand 10 minutes. Serve warm or cold.

GRANOLA SNACK BREAD

¾ C. all-purpose flour
½ C. granulated sugar
½ tsp. baking powder
½ tsp. salt
¼ tsp. ground allspice
½ C. egg substitute
⅓ C. margarine

⅓ C. skim milk
⅓ C. packed brown sugar
2 tsp. cornstarch
⅓ C. evaporated skim milk
2 tsp. safflower oil
½ C. granola
3 T. raisins

In a large mixer bowl, combine the flour, sugar, baking powder, salt and allspice; mix well. Add the egg substitute, margarine and milk. Beat until well combined; beat for about 2 minutes on medium speed. Turn batter into an 8x1½" round microwave-safe baking dish coated lightly with vegetable oil cooking spray. Microwave, uncovered, on MEDIUM (50% power) for 9 to 10 minutes or until cake tests almost done; turn dish a quarter-turn every 3 minutes. Microwave, uncovered, on HIGH (100% power) for 1 to 1½ minutes or until wooden pick inserted in center comes out clean. Let cake stand 5 minutes. In a small microwave-safe bowl, combine the brown sugar and cornstarch. Stir in the evaporated milk and oil. Microwave on HIGH for 1½ to 2 minutes or until mixture is thick and bubbly, stirring every 30 seconds. Stir in granola and raisins. Spread over top of bread. Serve warm.

MEXICAN CHICKEN TACOS

⅓ C. chopped green pepper
1½ C. cubed cooked chicken
1 C. taco sauce
8 taco shells
2¼ C. chopped fresh
  spinach

½ C. shredded lowfat
  Cheddar cheese
½ C. chopped tomato (1 sm.)
¼ C. chopped ripe olives

In 1-quart microwave-safe bowl, microwave, covered, on HIGH (100% power), the green pepper for 1½ minutes or until tender-crisp. Stir in chicken and taco sauce. Cover; microwave on HIGH for 3 to 3½ minutes or until heated. Spoon ¼ cup chicken mixture into each taco shell. Top with ¼ cup spinach, 1 tablespoon each of tomato and cheese and ½ tablespoon olives. Makes 8 tacos.

ORANGE CHICKEN STRIPS
WITH RICE AND BROCCOLI

2 tsp. margarine
12 oz. skinless, boneless
  chicken breast
Garlic salt
1 C. quick-cooking rice

1 C. hot water
2 C. frozen broccoli
¼ tsp. ground ginger
1½ T. frozen orange juice
  concentrate

In a 10x6'' microwave-safe baking dish, microwave on HIGH (100% power) the margarine for 30 to 60 seconds or until melted. Cut chicken into strips. Add to margarine and coat evenly. Sprinkle with garlic salt. Microwave on HIGH for 4 to 5 minutes or until chicken is no longer pink, stirring once. Add rice, water, broccoli and ginger; mix lightly. Cover with plastic wrap and microwave on HIGH 8 to 10 minutes or until rice is tender. Stir in concentrate and serve. Makes 4 servings.

PINEAPPLE-PEANUT LAMB CHOPS

¾ C. quick-cooking rice
¾ C. water
1 (8¼ oz.) can crushed
  pineapple
¼ C. chopped peanuts
¼ C. sliced green onions

Dash ground cloves
4 lamb leg sirloin chops
  (cut ¾" thick, 1¼ lbs.)
1 T. soy sauce (low-salt)
2 tsp. cornstarch

In a 1-quart microwave-safe casserole, combine the rice and water. Microwave, covered, on HIGH (100% power) for 3 to 5 minutes or until the water is boiling. Let stand, covered, 5 minutes. Meanwhile, drain crushed pineapple over a 1-cup measure. Measure juice. Add water, if necessary, to equal $\frac{1}{3}$ cup. Set juice aside. In an 8x8x2'' microwave-safe baking dish, combine drained pineapple, peanuts, half of the green onions and cloves. Stir in the hot cooked rice. Spread rice mixture in the baking dish. Trim fat from lamb. Sprinkle with pepper. Arrange chops atop rice mixture with the meatiest portions toward the outside of the dish. Cover with waxed paper. Cook on HIGH for 8 to 11 minutes or until done, turning chops over and rearranging once. Meanwhile, for sauce, stir remaining green onion, soy sauce and cornstarch into reserved pineapple juice. Cook, uncovered, on HIGH for $1\frac{1}{2}$ to $2\frac{1}{2}$ minutes or until thickened and bubbly, stirring every 30 seconds. Serve sauce over meat. If desired, garnish with a green onion brush. Makes 4 servings.

NUTRITIOUS POPCORN

2 qts. popped popcorn
1 C. salted peanuts
1 C. sunflower kernels
⅓ C. sugar
¼ C. margarine

1 tsp. ground cinnamon
½ C. honey
¾ C. raisins
¾ C. snipped dried apricots

In a 12" square microwave-safe baking dish, combine popcorn, peanuts and sunflower kernels; mix well. Set aside. In a 1-quart microwave-safe measure, combine sugar, margarine and cinnamon. Drizzle honey over sugar mixture. Microwave on HIGH (100% power) for 2 minutes; stir well. Microwave on MEDIUM-LOW (30% power) for 5 minutes, stirring once. Pour over popcorn mixture. Mix well, coating all pieces with syrup. Microwave popcorn mixture on MEDIUM-LOW for 5 minutes, stirring once. Add raisins and apricots; mix well. Cool completely and store in a tightly covered container. Makes 12 cups.

70

RHUBARB SAUCE

2¼ C. chopped rhubarb

2 T. water
½ C. sugar

In a 2-quart microwave-safe casserole, combine the rhubarb and water. Microwave, covered, on HIGH (100% power) for 3 to 4 minutes or until rhubarb is tender, stirring once during cook time. Add sugar and mix well. Microwave on HIGH for 1 minute or until sugar is dissolved. Cool, covered. Maybe served warm or cold. Makes 2 cups sauce.

WHOLE WHEAT CHIPS

1 C. whole wheat flour   ¼ C. margarine
2 tsp. sesame seed   3 to 4 T. cold water

In mixing bowl, combine flour and sesame seed. Cut in margarine at low speed until particles resemble cornmeal (a pastry blender may also be used). Sprinkle water, 1 tablespoon at a time, over mixture; stir with a fork after each addition. Use just enough water until dough is moist enough to hold together. Form dough into a square, flattening to ½" thickness. On floured pastry cloth, roll out dough to a 14x12" rectangle; smooth or trim edges. Cut into 2" squares. Arrange 11 at a time, close together, around edge of a large microwave-safe pie plate coated lightly with vegetable oil cooking spray. Microwave on HIGH (100% power) 2 to 6 minutes or until dry and firm; rotate ½ turn after 1 minute and check often. Remove carefully and transfer to wire rack. Chips will crisp as they cool Makes 3½ dozen.

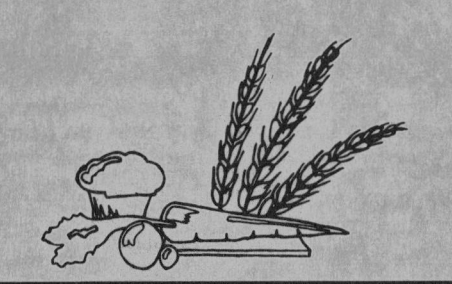

VEGETABLES

APPLES AND CABBAGE

COMBINE IN A PAN:
2 C. shredded cabbage   *¼ C. hot water*
1 apple (chopped)   *½ tsp. salt*
¼ C. cider vinegar   *2 T. sugar*

Cook, tightly covered, until tender. Serves 4.

ASPARAGUS AND CORN CASSEROLE

1 pkg. frozen corn
1 lb. can asparagus or fresh
 cooked asparagus
2 T. margarine
2 T. flour

½ C. milk, skim
¼ tsp. celery salt
1 C. margined bread crumbs
 or oat bran
2 T. grated Parmesan cheese

Cook corn until barely tender, drain, and reserve liquid. Drain asparagus and reserve liquid. Melt margarine in saucepan and blend in flour. Gradually add milk, vegetable liquids (½ cup). Stir until thick and smooth. Add celery salt. Layer corn and asparagus in a sprayed casserole. Pour cream sauce over that and top with bran or crumbs and cheese. Bake at 350° for 20 minutes.

BAKED BEAN CASSEROLE

2 T. oil
1½ C. thinly sliced onions
1½ C. thinly sliced green
  peppers
2 (1 lb. ea.) cans vegetarian
  baked beans

2 C. diced tomatoes
⅛ tsp. salt
⅓ tsp. freshly ground black
  pepper

Saute onion and peppers in oiled skillet. In a casserole arrange successive layers of the beans, tomatoes and sauteed vegetables. Sprinkle vegetables with salt and pepper. Make a top layer of tomatoes. Bake at 350° for 30 minutes.

BAKED CARROTS

2 lbs. carrots
¼ C. (½ stick) melted
  margarine
1 T. sugar

¾ tsp. salt
¼ tsp. pepper
1 T. chopped parsley

Clean carrots and slice very thin or grate coarsely. Put carrots in a greased 1½-quart casserole. Sprinkle with margarine, sugar, salt and pepper. Toss lightly. Cover and bake in a preheated 350° oven for 40 to 50 minutes. Serve hot, garnished with parsley.

BAKED YAMS

3 lg. yams
2 T. margarine

Salt and pepper
Margarine

Wash yams and wipe dry; rub with margarine. Bake in preheated 400° oven for 1 hour or until potatoes feel soft when squeezed. Cut baked yams in half; cut crosswise slit in yams and squeeze. Serve hot with salt and pepper and additional margarine.

BROCCOLI GINGER STIR-FRY

2 T. oil
4 C. bite-size broccoli florets
2 garlic cloves (minced)

1 T. low sodium soy sauce
1 tsp. minced gingerroot

Heat large skillet or wok over medium-high heat until hot. Add oil and heat until it ripples. Add broccoli, garlic, soy sauce and gingerroot. Stir-fry for 2 to 4 minutes or until broccoli is crisp-tender. Serves 8 (½ cup each).

BULGUR AND VEGETABLES

1¾ C. water
⅓ C. chopped onion
1 tsp. low-sodium bouillon
  granules
1 clove garlic (minced)
1 C. sliced fresh
  mushrooms (3 oz.)
1 sm. zucchini (quartered
  lengthwise and sliced)

1 med. tomato (chopped)
1 C. bulgur
¼ C. chopped green pepper
⅓ C. sliced carrot
½ tsp. dried basil (crushed)
½ tsp. celery seed
¼ tsp. dried thyme or
  marjoram (crushed)

In a medium saucepan combine water, onion, bouillon granules and garlic; simmer until tender. Stir in remaining ingredients and ¼ teaspoon pepper. Bring to boiling; reduce heat. Cover; simmer for 15 to 20 minutes or until bulgur is tender. Makes 4 servings.

CHINESE STYLE CABBAGE

1 T. oil
3 C. finely shredded cabbage
1 C. celery (chopped)
1 green pepper (chopped)

1 onion (chopped)
½ tsp. salt or less
⅛ tsp. pepper

Heat oil in skillet. Drop in vegetables and stir well. Cover tightly and steam for 5 minutes, stirring several times. Season with salt and pepper. Serve immediately. May top with soy sauce (low-sodium).

CORN AND GREEN BEANS

1 C. fresh or frozen French-
style green beans
1 C. frozen whole kernel
corn or fresh (cut from cob)
½ C. water

1 T. margarine
3 T. chopped onion
½ tsp. lemon juice
Dash pepper
½ tsp. basil

Cook beans and corn together in water until beans are just tender. Drain. In a separate pan, cook onion in margarine until tender. Pour over beans and corn and add basil, lemon juice and pepper. Simmer until hot (VARIATION: Succotosh - Use fresh lima beans in place of green beans.) Makes 4 servings.

EGGPLANT HOT DISH

1½ C. canned garbanzo beans
  (drained and rinsed) or
  1 pkg. baby limas (thawed)
Olive oil
2 med. eggplants

½ tsp. salt
Black pepper
4 C. chopped and drained
  tomatoes

Peel and slice eggplants. Sprinkle with salt and let stand for 1 hour. Drain and cube. Brown in olive oil. Add rest of ingredients and bake in 2-quart casserole for 40 minutes at 350°. Makes 6 to 8 servings.

FRENCH GREEN PEAS

1 C. shredded lettuce
2 pkgs. frozen tiny green
  peas (thawed)
4 green onions (sliced)

2 T. margarine
¼ tsp. salt
½ tsp. sugar
3 T. water

Mix ingredients in a saucepan; cover and cook over low heat for 25 minutes. Drain.

FRESH SWEET AND SOUR BEANS

3 C. chicken stock
16 oz. fresh green beans
1 tsp. mild soy sauce
1 sliced carrot
3 T. apple cider vinegar

¼ C. unbleached flour
¼ C. sm. onion (grated)
¼ C. frozen unsweetened
  apple juice concentrate

Add green beans, soy sauce and carrot to boiling stock, cover and simmer 1 to 1½ hours, or until beans are tender. Brown flour in a heavy skillet, stirring constantly with a wooden spoon until golden brown. Remove from heat, add grated onion and blend. Add browned flour mixture to cooked beans and blend. Add apple juice concentrate and vinegar, and stir over low heat until a smooth sauce results. Simmer 20 minutes. Taste, and adjust seasonings. May be prepared the day before and reheated for serving.

MICROWAVED VEGETABLE ORIENTAL

The basics of stir-frying are replaced by the magic of microwave cooking.

12 oz. fresh Chinese pea
    pods (washed and strings
    and ends removed), plus
2 T. water
1 C. sliced fresh mushrooms
4 oz. water chestnuts (rinsed,
    drained and sliced)

2 oz. chopped pimiento
    (drained)
½ tsp. garlic powder
½ C. sliced green onions
1½ C. fresh bean sprouts
¼ C. water or chicken stock
4 tsp. mild soy sauce

Place pea pods and the 2 tablespoons water in a 3-quart covered casserole. Microwave on HIGH for 2 minutes. Stir and microwave 2 additional minutes. Add remaining ingredients to pea pods, mix gently, cover and microwave on HIGH 1 to 2 minutes, or until crisp.

REFRIED BEANS

2 C. cooked drained pinto
  beans
¼ C. finely chopped onions
⅛ tsp. garlic powder

⅛ tsp. hot pepper sauce
¼ tsp. chili powder
½ C. oil
½ C. shredded lowfat sharp
  Cheddar

Mash beans until almost smooth. Combine with onions, garlic powder, hot sauce and chili powder; mix to blend. Heat oil in heavy frying pan over moderate heat and add bean mixture; cook and stir over moderate heat until beans turn dark and edges are crisp and brown. Sprinkle with cheese and stir gently until cheese is melted. Serve hot. Serves 4 to 6 servings.

SAUTEED CAULIFLOWER

1 head (1 lb.) fresh or 1
  (10 oz.) pkg. frozen
  cauliflower
2 T. oil
¼ tsp. thyme
¾ tsp. vinegar

½ garlic clove (minced)
Dash pepper
2 tsp. minced parsley or
  1 tsp. dry parsley flakes

Break the cauliflower into small flowerettes and cook or steam in unsalted water until just tender, 10 to 12 minutes; or cook frozen cauliflower according to directions on package. Drain. Combine and heat oil, thyme, vinegar and garlic in a large pan or skillet over moderate heat 5 minutes. Add drained cauliflower, sprinkle with pepper and stir gently. Simmer until hot. Sprinkle with parsley before serving. Serves 4.

SHREDDED CARROTS

1½ lbs. carrots
3 T. margarine

Salt and pepper to taste

Clean carrots and shred coarsely. Melt margarine in frying pan. Spread carrots evenly in frying pan; cover tightly and cook over moderate heat for 4 minutes. Turn with a pancake turner, cover tightly, and cook about 4 to 5 minutes longer; the cooking time depends upon the tenderness of the carrots. Serve hot, seasoned with salt and pepper. Serves 4 to 6.

SOUTHERN BLACK-EYED PEAS

1 lb. dried black-eyed peas
1½ qts. water
4 oz. bacon

Hot water
Salt and pepper
Corn bread

Pick over peas, removing any dark or discolored ones. Add peas to 1½ quarts water in a heavy saucepan; bring to a boil and cook 2 minutes. Remove from heat, cover and let stand 1½ to 2 hours. Return peas to heat and add bacon; cover and cook about 1½ hours or until tender, adding hot water, if necessary, to keep the peas covered with liquid. Add salt and pepper to taste. Serve hot; it is customary to serve this dish with corn bread.

SPICY CABBAGE DISH

3 slices bacon, chopped
¾ C. tomato juice
¾ C. beef bouillon
¼ tsp. garlic powder

¼ tsp. oregano
½ tsp. salt (optional)
⅛ tsp. pepper
2 lb. head cabbage

Fry chopped bacon over medium heat in a heavy saucepan until crisp; add tomato juice, bouillon, garlic powder, oregano, salt and pepper. Cover and cook 5 minutes over medium heat. Clean cabbage and chop coarsely or shred; add cabbage to sauce. Cover and cook 12 minutes over medium heat, stirring occasionally.

SUCCOTASH

1-10 oz. pkg. frozen lima
   beans
1-10 oz. pkg. frozen whole-
   kernel corn
2 T. melted margarine

⅛ tsp. pepper
1 T. chopped parsley

Cook vegetables in salted water according to package directions; drain well. Combine vegetables with margarine, pepper and parsley. Serve hot.

STIR-FRY BROCCOLI

2 bunches broccoli, flowers
  only
4 T. peanut oil

1 can water chestnuts (diced)
1 lb. lean, cubed beef

SEASONING SAUCE:
1 tsp. salt-free herb
  seasoning
½ tsp. salt

1 tsp. sugar
½ C. chicken broth
  (low sodium)

THICKENING SAUCE:
1 T. cornstarch
2 tsp. soy sauce (low
  sodium)

3 T. water

Cook broccoli for 2 to 3 minutes; drain. Heat oil and brown meat. Add water chestnuts and cook for 2 to 3 minutes. Add broccoli and seasoning sauce. Cook for several minutes. Add thickening sauce and cook until thick. Serve over meat and rice.

SWEET POTATO FRITTERS

4 sweet potatoes, pared,
  cooked, and mashed,
  (about 2 to 2½ C.)
2 well-beaten eggs
1 T. softened margarine

½ C. skim milk
¼ C. flour
1 tsp. ground allspice
1 tsp. salt (optional)
½ C. chopped
  English walnuts

Mix sweet potatoes and eggs; add margarine and milk and beat 1 minute at medium speed. Add flour, allspice and salt; mix 1 minute at medium speed. Add walnuts and mix ½ minute at medium speed or until well blended. Drop by tablespoonfuls into preheated 365° deep fat fryer; fry 2 to 3 minutes, turning several times until fritters are golden brown. Remove from fat with slotted spoon and drain over hot fat, place on paper toweling. Serve hot. Fritters can be kept hot for a short time in a warm oven until the whole batch is ready.

SWEET-SOUR CABBAGE

1 med. size head red cabbage
2 C. cold water
1 tsp. salt
½ C. sliced onion
¼ C. (½ stick) margarine
¼ C. brown sugar

2 T. flour
½ C. water
¼ C. vinegar
¾ tsp. salt
⅛ tsp. pepper

Clean, core and shred cabbage. Put the cabbage with 2 cups cold water and 1 teaspoon salt in a heavy saucepan, cover and cook for 8 to 10 minutes. Cook the onions in margarine until golden. Add the sugar, flour, water, vinegar, salt and pepper to the onions. Cook and stir until smooth and thickened. Drain cabbage and add it to thickened sauce; mix well. Heat the cabbage through. Garnish with bacon bits. Serves 4 to 6.

VEGETABLES IN COMBO

2 C. sliced fresh green beans
1 med. onion (cut into wedges)
2 C. sliced zucchini

2 C. sliced summer squash
2 lg. tomatoes
  (cut into wedges)
Italian seasoning

In a large saucepan cook green beans and onions, covered, in a small amount of boiling water for 15 minutes. Add zucchini and summer squash. Cook, covered, for 5 to 10 minutes more or until vegetables are crisp-tender. Add tomatoes; heat through. To serve, sprinkle with Italian seasoning to taste. Makes 6 servings.

VEGETABLES WITH BASIL

1¼ C. fresh pea pods (strings and stems removed)
1 med. zucchini (thinly sliced)
1 T. margarine

1 T. snipped basil or 1 tsp. dried basil (crushed)
12 cherry tomatoes (halved)
1 T. toasted pine nuts or almonds

In a 2-quart saucepan cook the pea pods and zucchini in a small amount of boiling water for 2 minutes. Drain and set aside. In the same saucepan melt the margarine. Add the basil and cook for 1 to 2 minutes. Add the tomatoes, zucchini and pea pods. Lightly toss vegetables to coat with the margarine mixture. Heat through. Arrange the vegetables on individual serving plates; sprinkle with nuts. Season to taste. Makes 4 servings.

YAMS WITH PINEAPPLE

3½ C. yams without sugar
  syrup
1 C. crushed pineapple
  and juice

¾ C. brown sugar
¼ C. (½ stick) margarine
¼ tsp. salt
⅛ tsp. ground cinnamon

Drain yams well and spread in greased 9" square baking dish. Mix pineapple, brown sugar, margarine, salt and cinnamon at low speed for 1 minute or until blended; spread mixture evenly over yams. Bake in preheated 350° oven for 1 hour or until browned. Serve hot.

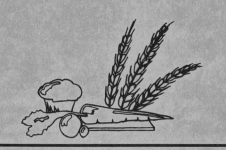

SALADS

APPLE, CABBAGE AND DATE SALAD

¼ C. salad dressing
1 T. skim milk
¼ tsp. salt
2 T. sugar

1 med.-size firm, red apple
½ C. chopped dates
½ C. miniature marshmallows
1 qt. shredded cabbage

Combine salad dressing, skim milk, salt and sugar in a mixing bowl; stir to blend well. Wash and core apple, and cut into thin, small wedges, adding to dressing mixture as you slice, mixing to coat the apple. Add dates, marshmallows and cabbage and toss lightly; refrigerate. Toss just before serving. Serves 6 to 8.

CARROT AND RAISIN SALAD

¾ C. washed and drained
   raisins
2 C. coarsely grated carrots
1 C. drained, canned
   pineapple tidbits (in own
   juice)

⅓ C. salad dressing
1 T. lemon juice
¼ tsp. salt (optional)
1 T. sugar

Toss raisins, carrots and pineapple together lightly, add dressing made by stirring salad dressing lemon juice, salt and sugar together. Refrigerate until served.

CHILI BEAN SALAD

1 ½ lbs. fresh green beans or
2 (9 oz. ea.) pkgs. frozen
  beans
15 oz. can garbanzo beans
  (drained)
¼ C. lemon juice
2 T. oil
½ tsp. chili powder

¼ tsp. salt
⅛ tsp. celery seed
1 clove garlic (minced)
Dash of red pepper
1 med. onion sliced and
  separated into rings

Cook green beans in salted water until tendercrisp; drain. Place green beans and garbanzo beans in large bowl or utility dish. Combine lemon juice, oil, chili powder, salt, celery seed, garlic and red pepper; cook slowly for 4 to 5 minutes. Add onion rings and continue cooking 2 to 3 minutes. Cool and pour over beans, stirring lightly to combine. Cover and marinate in refrigerator for 3 to 4 hours or overnight. Serve cold or heat and serve hot, if desired. Makes 8 servings.

CITRUS MARINATED FRUIT

FRUIT:
1 C. cantaloupe balls or cubes
1 C. blueberries
1 C. halved or whole strawberries

1 C. halved seedless
green grapes

ORANGE MARMALADE:
1 T. sugar
¾ C. orange juice
2 T. lemon juice

¼ C. white grape juice or dry
white wine
Fresh mint leaves (if desired)

In large bowl, combine fruit. In small bowl, combine all marinade ingredients except mint leaves; mix well. Pour marinade over fruit. Cover and refrigerate for 2 to 3 hours to blend flavors, stirring occasionally. To serve, spoon fruit and marinade into individual dishes. Garnish with mint leaves. Serves 8 (½ cup each).

102

COLESLAW VINAIGRETTE WITH GRAPES

½ C. cider vinegar
2 T. sugar
2 tsp. Dijon-type mustard

1 tsp. freshly ground pepper
⅔ C. salad oil

2 sm. heads (about 1 lb. ea.)
  cabbage (red or white)
¼ C. chopped parsley
3 T. chopped green onion

¼ C. toasted pine nuts or
  slivered almonds
1 to 1½ C. seedless grapes
  (red or green or
  a combination)

In small bowl or jar blend vinegar, sugar, mustard, pepper and oil. Set aside. Shred cabbage finely, place in large bowl and combine with parsley and green onions; toss with dressing. Cover and refrigerate 1 to 6 hours. When ready to serve, drain off extra dressing and spoon coleslaw into chilled bowl. Top with toasted nuts and grapes. Makes 10 servings.   103

CORN SALAD

2 C. drained, canned whole
   kernel corn
¼ C. chopped pimentos
½ C. chopped fresh green
   peppers

¼ C. finely chopped onions
¼ C. diced cucumbers
¾ C. French dressing

Mix the corn, pimientos, green peppers, onions and cucumbers. Add the
French dressing and toss the salad. Refrigerate for 1 to 3 hours. Drain and
toss salad before serving.

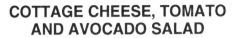

COTTAGE CHEESE, TOMATO AND AVOCADO SALAD

1 qt. (2 lbs.) lowfat cottage
  cheese
2 peeled and diced
  medium-sized tomatoes
⅔ C. chopped fresh green
  peppers

¼ tsp. dill weed
8 peeled avocado halves
Salad greens
½ C. chopped roasted
  peanuts or toasted almonds

Combine cheese, tomatoes, green peppers and dill; chill at least 30 minutes. Arrange avocado halves on salad greens, mound cheese mixture on top and sprinkle with chopped nuts. Serve with whole-wheat bread.

CUCUMBER SALAD

Dissolve 1 package lemon gelatin in 1½ cups boiling water. When cool add:

¼ C. finely chopped celery
¼ C. finely chopped green
    pepper

1 C. grated cucumber
1 onion (grated)

Put into a mold and chill until firm. Serve on crisp greens. Serves 4.

KIDNEY BEAN SALAD

⅓ C. salad dressing
½ tsp. salt (optional)
1 T. lemon juice
2 C. (1 lb. can) washed
  and drained cooked
  kidney beans
4 chopped hard-cooked
  eggs

¾ C. thinly sliced celery
¼ C. finely chopped onions
⅓ C. drained sweet
  pickle relish
4 oz. diced lowfat American
  process or Cheddar cheese
1 T. chopped pimiento

Mix salad dressing, salt and lemon juice and add to beans; mix lightly to coat beans with dressing. Add eggs, celery, onions, relish, cheese and pimiento and toss lightly. Refrigerate until served.

MACARONI SLAW

1 C. uncooked elbow macaroni	1½ C. finely chopped or shredded cabbage
½ C. salad dressing	½ C. coarsely chopped or shredded carrots
1 T. lemon juice	
2 tsp. sugar	⅓ C. finely chopped fresh green peppers
1 tsp. prepared mustard	
¼ tsp. salt	⅓ C. finely chopped onions
⅛ tsp. garlic powder	

Cook macaroni according to package directions; you should have about 3 cups of cooked macaroni. Rinse with cold water and drain well; stir to separate pieces. Stir salad dressing, lemon juice, sugar, mustard, salt and garlic powder together to form a dressing. Add cabbage, carrots, peppers, onions and salad dressing to macaroni; mix lightly. Refrigerate until served. Makes 1 quart.

MELON CUP

2 C. watermelon balls
2 C. cantaloupe balls
2 C. honeydew balls

4 T. orange-flavored liqueur
 or thawed frozen orange
 juice concentrate

In a glass serving dish, combine melon balls. Drizzle with liqueur. Cover and refrigerate until chilled. To serve, stir gently. Makes 4 to 6 servings.

MUSHROOM-ORANGE SALAD

⅓ C. special oil
1 T. sugar
⅛ tsp. salt
3 T. vinegar
4.5 oz. jar sliced mushrooms
  (drained)

4 C. torn romaine lettuce
⅓ C. raisins
¼ C. sliced green onions
11 oz. can mandarin orange
  segments (drained)

In a large bowl, blend oil, sugar, salt and vinegar. Stir in mushrooms and refrigerate at least 1 hour. Just before serving, add remaining ingredients and toss gently.

PRUNE PLUM SALAD

2 C. (1 lb. can) prune plums
Water
1-3 oz. pkg. cherry flavored
  gelatin

1 C. boiling water
¾ C. miniature marshmallows

Drain and pit prune plums. Measure juice and add enough water, if necessary, to yield 1 cup liquid. Dissolve gelatin in boiling water; add plum juice and water. Refrigerate until slightly thickened. Stir pitted plums and marshmallows into gelatin and pour into a 1-quart mold rinsed with cold water. Chill until firm. Serves 4 to 6.

THREE-BEAN SALAD

1 C. cooked, drained green
string beans, cut into
1" lengths
1 C. cooked, drained yellow
wax beans, cut into
1" lengths
1 C. washed and drained
cooked red kidney beans

¼ C. thinly sliced
sweet onions
⅓ C. chopped fresh
green peppers
2 T. sliced pimiento-stuffed
green olives
French or Italian style vinegar
and oil dressing

Combine beans, onion, green peppers and olives; toss lightly with dressing, as desired. Refrigerate 4 hours or overnight and toss salad just before serving.

TROPICAL FRUIT SALAD

2 bananas
1 T. lemon juice
2 kiwifruits, peeled, cut
  crosswise in ¼" slices
1 (15¼ oz.) can pineapple
  slices (juice pack) , drained,
  cut in halves
1 pt. strawberries

1 papaya, if desired,
  cut in quarters
1 caramabola, if desired,
  sliced crosswise
  in ¼" slices
¼ C. papaya nectar
2 tsp. honey
½ C. plain lowfat yogurt

Peel and cut bananas in half crosswise, then cut each half lengthwise. In a medium-size bowl, gently toss bananas with lemon juice. Arrange fruits on a large platter. To make dressing, in a small bowl, stir nectar and honey until honey dissolves; mix in yogurt. Pour dressing over salad. Makes 6 servings.

TOSSED TURKEY AND BERRIES

1 pt. fresh strawberries
4 C. torn mixed greens
¼ C. red wine vinegar and
  oil salad dressing
½ of a sweet red onion
  (sliced, separated into rings
  and halved)

¾ lb. turkey breast tenderloin
  steaks or skinless, boneless
  chicken breasts
  (cut into bite-size strips)
2 T. honey
¾ tsp. snipped fresh dill
  weed or ¼ tsp. dried
  dill weed)

Hull strawberries and discard the hulls. Halve strawberries. In a large mixing bowl combine strawberries and mixed greens. Set aside. In a 12" skillet heat half of the salad dressing. Add the red onion. Stir-fry for 1½ to 2 minutes or until onion is tender. Remove from the skillet. Heat the remaining dressing in same skillet. Stir-fry the turkey or chicken in the hot dressing for 2 to 3 minutes or until done. Add onion, honey and dill weed; heat through. Remove the skillet from heat. Immediately add greens mixture; lightly toss about 1 minute or until greens begin to wilt. Serve at once. Season with salt and pepper. Serves 4.

YELLOW WAX BEAN SALAD

3 C. cold cooked, drained
   yellow wax beans cut into
   1" lengths
⅓ C. diced fresh green
   peppers

⅓ C. thinly sliced
   sweet onions
Italian vinegar
   and oil dressing

Toss beans, green peppers, onion, and salad dressing, as desired, together; serve at room temperature. Yields: 4 to 6 servings.

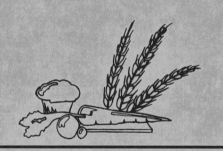

DESSERTS

APPLESAUCE AND BRAN BAKE

3 lg. green cooking apples
1 C. water
¼ C. date "sugar" or
* fructose*

4 tsp. unprocessed oat bran
½ tsp. ground cinnamon
¼ tsp. ground nutmeg
½ tsp. vanilla extract

Preheat oven to 325°. Dice apples into 1" cubes, removing the core completely. Mix all other ingredients in the water. Place the diced apples in a glass loaf pan or baking dish. Pour the water mixture over the apples. Bake, uncovered, in the preheated oven for 45 minutes. Remove from oven and allow baked apples to come to room temperature. Store in the refrigerator. This applesauce is an excellent accompaniment to many meats. It's a good breakfast fruit, a light dessert and the basic ingredient for Applesauce Topping. If you prefer a smooth, creamy applesauce, put the baked apples and all the cooking liquid in a blender and blend until smooth. If necessary add ¼ cup more water to make a creamier consistency. Yields: 2 cups.

BANANA OATMEAL COOKIES

3 bananas
⅓ C. vegetable oil
2 C. rolled oats
1½ C. chopped dates

½ C. chopped walnuts
1 tsp. vanilla extract
¼ tsp. salt

In a large bowl, mash the bananas and add the remaining ingredients. Mix well and drop by rounded tablespoons onto a non-stick cookie sheet. Bake for 20 to 25 minutes in a preheated 350° oven. Remove to wire rack to cool.

BRAN PEANUT BUTTER COOKIES

1 C. margarine
¾ C. granulated sugar
¾ C. brown sugar (firmly
  packed)
½ C. egg substitute
¾ C. peanut butter

1 tsp. vanilla extract
1¼ C. all-purpose flour
1 C. 100% Bran
¾ C. uncooked quick oats
2 tsp. baking soda
½ tsp. salt

Preheat oven to 350°. In bowl, with electric mixer at medium speed, beat margarine, granulated sugar and brown sugar for 3 minutes or until light and fluffy. Beat in egg substitute, peanut butter and vanilla extract. In medium bowl, combine flour, 100% Bran, oats, baking soda and salt; gradually add to peanut butter mixture; beat until well combined. Drop by tablespoonfuls onto ungreased cookie sheets; bake for 12 to 15 minutes or until lightly browned.

BRAN PIE CRUST

¾ C. whole wheat pastry flour   ¼ C. corn oil
¼ C. unprocessed oat bran   3 T. ice water
¼ tsp. salt

Preheat the oven to 375°. Put flour, bran and salt in a 9" pie pan and mix well. Measure the oil in a measuring cup. Add the water to the oil and mix well, using a fork. Slowly add the liquid to the flour-bran mixture in the pie pan, mixing it with the same fork. Continue mixing until all ingredients are well blended. Press it into shape with your fingers, making sure it covers the entire inner surface of the pie pan evenly. Prick the bottom of the crust with a fork and place in a 375° oven for 20 minutes if the recipe you are using calls for a prebaked pie crust. Makes 1-9" crust.

BRAN-DATE CUPCAKES

1½ C. chopped dates
¾ tsp. baking soda
¾ C. boiling water
¼ C. oil
¾ C. sugar

½ tsp. vanilla extract
1½ C. sifted flour
½ C. bran flakes
½ C. chopped walnuts

Mix the dates and baking soda; mix in the boiling water and let cool. Blend the oil, sugar and vanilla. Beat in the flour, bran and nuts. Spoon into 12 oiled muffin pans. Bake at 350°.

CARROT CAKE

1½ C. peanut oil
2 C. granulated sugar
1 C. egg substitute
5 T. hot water
2½ C. all-purpose flour
1½ tsp. baking powder
½ tsp. baking soda
¼ tsp. salt

1 tsp. ground cinnamon
1 tsp. ground cloves
½ tsp. ground nutmeg
1¾ C. grated raw carrots
1 C. 100% Bran
1 (2¼ oz.) bag pecan pieces
 (chopped)
Confectioners' sugar

Preheat oven to 350°. Grease bottom and sides of large bundt pan. In a small bowl combine water and bran; set aside. In large bowl, with electric mixer at low speed, blend, peanut oil and sugar. Add egg substitute, beating well. In medium bowl, combine flour, baking powder, baking soda, salt, cinnamon, cloves and nutmeg. Gradually add to sugar mixture, beating well after each addition. Stir in carrots, Bran and pecans. Pour into prepared pan. Bake for 60 to 70 minutes or until toothpick inserted 1" from center comes out clean. Cool in pan for 15 minutes; invert onto wire rack to cool completely. Sprinkle with confectioners' sugar.

CARROT COOKIES

1 C. margarine
¾ C. sugar
¼ C. egg substitute
1 C. cooked mashed carrots
2 C. flour

2 tsp. baking powder
1 tsp. vanilla
½ tsp. lemon extract
Dash of salt

Cream margarine and sugar. Add egg substitute, carrots and sifted flour with baking powder and salt added. Then add flavoring and drop by small teaspoon on oiled baking sheet. Frost while warm with icing made of the juice of 1 orange, ½ tablespoon orange peel and powdered sugar needed for desired thickness.

COCOA OAT BROWNIES

½ C. margarine
2 egg whites
1 tsp. vanilla
1 tsp. orange peel
1 tsp. lemon peel
1 C. pitted, chopped dates
⅓ C. cocoa
1 C. rolled oats

½ C. pastry flour
½ C. wheat germ
1 tsp. baking powder
½ tsp. ground allspice
½ tsp. nutmeg
½ tsp. cinnamon
⅔ C. skim milk

Combine margarine and egg whites; beat well. Add vanilla, orange peel, lemon peel, dates and cocoa; combine thoroughly. In a separate bowl, stir together oats, flour, wheat germ, baking powder and three spices. Combine two mixes, add milk and beat until blended. Spread batter in a 10x15'' rimmed baking dish. Sprinkle with nuts. Bake at 325° for 25 minutes. Cool on rack and cut into squares. Yield: 2 dozen.

DATE-BRAN COOKIES

½ C. margarine
1 C. brown sugar
1 egg or 2 egg whites
1 tsp. vanilla
1 C. all-purpose flour

½ tsp. baking soda
½ tsp. baking powder
½ C. chopped dates
2 C. 40% bran flakes

Cream margarine and brown sugar together until light and fluffy: Add egg or egg whites and vanilla and mix well. Stir flour, soda, baking powder and dates together until dates are separated and coated with flour mixture. Add with bran flakes to creamed mixture and stir only until flour is moistened. Drop by heaping tablespoonfuls onto lightly greased cookie sheets. Bake in preheated 375° oven for 15 minutes or until lightly browned. Remove cookies from pan while still warm. Makes 3 dozen cookies.

DELICIOUS BRAN BROWNIES

3 T. cocoa powder
1 T. instant coffee
1 T. water
2 ripe bananas
1½ C. sugar

6 egg whites
1 tsp. vanilla extract
1 C. oat-bran cereal
1 C. chopped pecans

Mix cocoa, water, coffee and bananas; put in a blender. Add the sugar, egg whites and vanilla; mix well. Add oat-bran cereal to the mixture. Fold in the nuts. Pour into a 9" baking pan sprayed with spray shortening or an oil and flour mixture. Bake at 350° for 45 minutes. Cut into individual squares, cool and serve.

EASY PEANUT BUTTER BARS

1 C. honey
1 C. peanut butter
½ C. cocoa
1 C. sesame seeds

1 C. sunflower seeds
½ C. coconut (shredded, optional)
½ C. chopped dates

Mix honey and peanut butter and beat over low heat. Add cocoa powder and mix well. Add rest of ingredients. Mix and pour into 9x9" pan and cool in refrigerator until hard. Cut into pieces.

FRESH RASPBERRY CRISP

1 qt. fresh raspberries
⅓ C. white sugar
¼ C. margarine
⅓ C. flour
⅓ C. brown sugar
¾ C. rolled oats

Place raspberries in bottom of a 9" square Pyrex cake pan and sprinkle with the white sugar. Blend margarine, flour, brown sugar and rolled oats until it resembles a coarse meal. Sprinkle the flour mixture over the raspberries and bake in a preheated moderate oven (350°) for about 30 minutes, or until lightly browned.

GOOD MORNING COOKIES

¾ C. margarine (softened)
⅓ C. honey
¼ C. brown sugar (packed)
½ C. egg substitute
1 tsp. vanilla
2 C. rolled oats
¾ C. whole wheat flour
⅓ C. unprocessed oat bran

½ tsp. baking soda
1 tsp. cinnamon
1 tsp. nutmeg
¼ tsp. salt (optional)
1 C. (about 6 oz.) pitted
prunes (chopped)
1 C. walnuts (chopped)

In mixer bowl, cream margarine, honey, sugar, egg substitute and vanilla. Combine oats, flour, oat bran, soda, cinnamon, nutmeg and salt; mix into creamed mixture. Stir in prunes and walnuts. Drop by generous spoonfuls onto two lightly greased baking sheets. Flatten to about ½". Bake at 350° for 15 minutes or until lightly browned. Cool on racks. Cookies can be frozen. Makes 12 breakfast cookies or 24 smaller cookies for snacking.   130

GRANDMA'S OLD-FASHIONED RICE PUDDING

1/3 C. raw short-grain brown
  rice (cooked 25 minutes in
  1 C. boiling water)
3¼ C. nonfat milk
¼ C. dry skim milk
½ C. frozen unsweetened
  apple juice concentrate
2 tsp. pure vanilla extract

4 egg whites (beaten just
  until foamy)
1 ripe banana (pureed)
⅔ C. muscat raisins
  (plumped 15 minutes in hot
  water to cover)
1 tsp. cinnamon
Freshly ground nutmeg
1 C. Grape-Nuts

Scald nonfat milk and dry skim milk. Add apple juice concentrate, vanilla, egg whites and pureed banana. Blend well. Place rice in a 1-quart oven-proof casserole or individual ramekins. Add raisins and cover with milk mixture. Sprinkle with Grape-Nuts, cinnamon and freshly ground nutmeg. Place casserole or ramekins in a baking dish with 1" of hot water and bake in a preheated 350° oven for 45 to 50 minutes. (When a sharp knife is inserted into custard, it should come out clean when pudding is done.)

OATMEAL DATE SQUARES

¾ C. pitted dates
1½ C. water
¾ C. sugar
1 C. margarine
2 C. brown sugar

2¼ C. rolled oats
2½ C. all-purpose flour
1½ tsp. baking soda
¾ tsp. salt
2 tsp. vanilla

Mix the dates, water and sugar in a heavy saucepan and cook over low heat, stirring constantly, until thick. Take the dates from the heat and cool. Blend the margarine, brown sugar, rolled oats, flour, soda, salt and vanilla; mix until it has a crumbly texture. Divide the oatmeal mixture in half. Spread half of the mixture evenly over the bottom of a greased 13x10" cake pan. Place date mixture into pan and spread over oatmeal mixture. Spread remaining half of oatmeal mixture over the filling and pat down so that it is smooth on top. Bake the squares in a preheated moderate oven (350°) for 25 to 30 minutes or until lightly browned. Cut into 6" squares while still warm. Makes 3 dozen.

OLD-FASHIONED PRUNE CAKE

1 C. sugar
½ C. shortening
2 eggs or 4 egg whites
1 C. all-purpose flour
1 C. graham flour
½ tsp. baking powder

½ tsp. ground cinnamon
½ tsp. ground cloves
1 tsp. baking soda
¼ C. sour milk
1 C. soaked, drained,
  chopped pitted
  unsweetened prunes

Cream sugar and shortening together until light and fluffy; add eggs and mix well. Stir flours, baking powder, cinnamon, cloves and soda together. Add flour mixture and milk to creamed mixture and beat 1 minute at medium speed; add prunes and beat 1 more minute at medium speed. Spread batter in a buttered 9x13" cake pan. Bake in a preheated 375° oven for 30 to 45 minutes or until done. Cool and frost in pan. Serve plain or with ice cream, if desired.

PEANUT BUTTER CAKE

1 C. sugar
½ C. shortening
1 C. smooth peanut butter
1 tsp. vanilla
3 eggs or 6 egg whites

1 C. all-purpose flour
1 C. graham flour
1 T. baking powder
½ tsp. salt
1 C. skim milk

Cream sugar, shortening, peanut butter and vanilla together until light and fluffy; add eggs and beat at medium speed for 2 minutes. Stir flours, baking powder and salt together to blend; add alternately with milk to creamed mixture and beat 1 minute at medium speed. Spread ½ of the batter in each of 2 greased and floured 9" layer cake pans. Bake in a preheated 375° oven for 35 to 40 minutes or until done. Cool 10 minutes in the pan; turn out on a wire rack to cool completely.

● ●

FILLING:
1 C. chopped dates
⅔ C. water
¼ C. sugar

⅛ tsp. salt
¼ C. crunchy peanut butter
Buttercream frosting

Cook and stir dates, water, sugar and salt over medium heat about 5 minutes or until thickened; remove from heat. Add peanut butter; cool to room temperature. Spread filling on 1 layer, cover with the remaining layer and frost with buttercream frosting.

PUMPKIN COOKIES

¼ C. margarine
½ C. sugar
1 egg or 2 egg whites
1 C. flour
2 tsp. baking powder
½ tsp. salt

1½ tsp. cinnamon
⅛ tsp. ginger
¼ tsp. nutmeg
½ C. cooked pumpkin
½ C. raisins
½ C. chopped nuts

Cream margarine and sugar until light. Add egg or whites and beat well. Sift dry ingredients and add to creamed mixture with the pumpkin. Mix well and add raisins and nuts. Drop from a teaspoon onto greased baking sheet. Bake at 375° for 15 minutes. Makes about 2 dozen medium sized cookies.

RAISIN CHIPPERS

2½ T. margarine
1 C. honey
1 tsp. vanilla
½ C. egg substitute

3 C. whole wheat flour
1 tsp. baking powder
1 (6 oz.) pkg. cocoa chips

Melt margarine over low heat and add honey, vanilla and lightly beaten egg substitute. Let cool. Combine flour and baking powder and add them to the cooled butter mixture. Stir in raisins and chips. Drop, teaspoon at a time on oiled cookie sheet, leaving space between to spread. Bake at 350° for 15 minutes. Yields: 24 cookies.

6 to 8 carrots (about 2 lbs.,
  thinly sliced)
½ C. water
½ C. orange juice
⅛ tsp. salt
½ C. sugar
½ C. egg substitute

¼ tsp. ground cinnamon
⅛ tsp. ground nutmeg
⅛ tsp. ground ginger
½ C. raisins
½ C. vanilla yogurt

Grease a 1½-quart souffle dish or deep steaming dish. In a small saucepan, combine carrots and water; cook over medium heat until tender. In a blender or food processor fitted with a metal blade, puree cooked carrots, any remaining cooking liquid and orange juice. Blend in salt, sugar, egg substitute, cinnamon, nutmeg and ginger. Stir in raisins. Spoon mixture into buttered dish. Place dish on a rack in a wok over simmering water; cover and steam 25 to 30 minutes or until firm and knife inserted off-center comes out clean. Refrigerate until chilled. Spoon into dessert dishes; top each serving with 1 tablespoon vanilla yogurt, if desired. Makes 8 servings.